The Employer's Business Case for Workplace Health Promotion

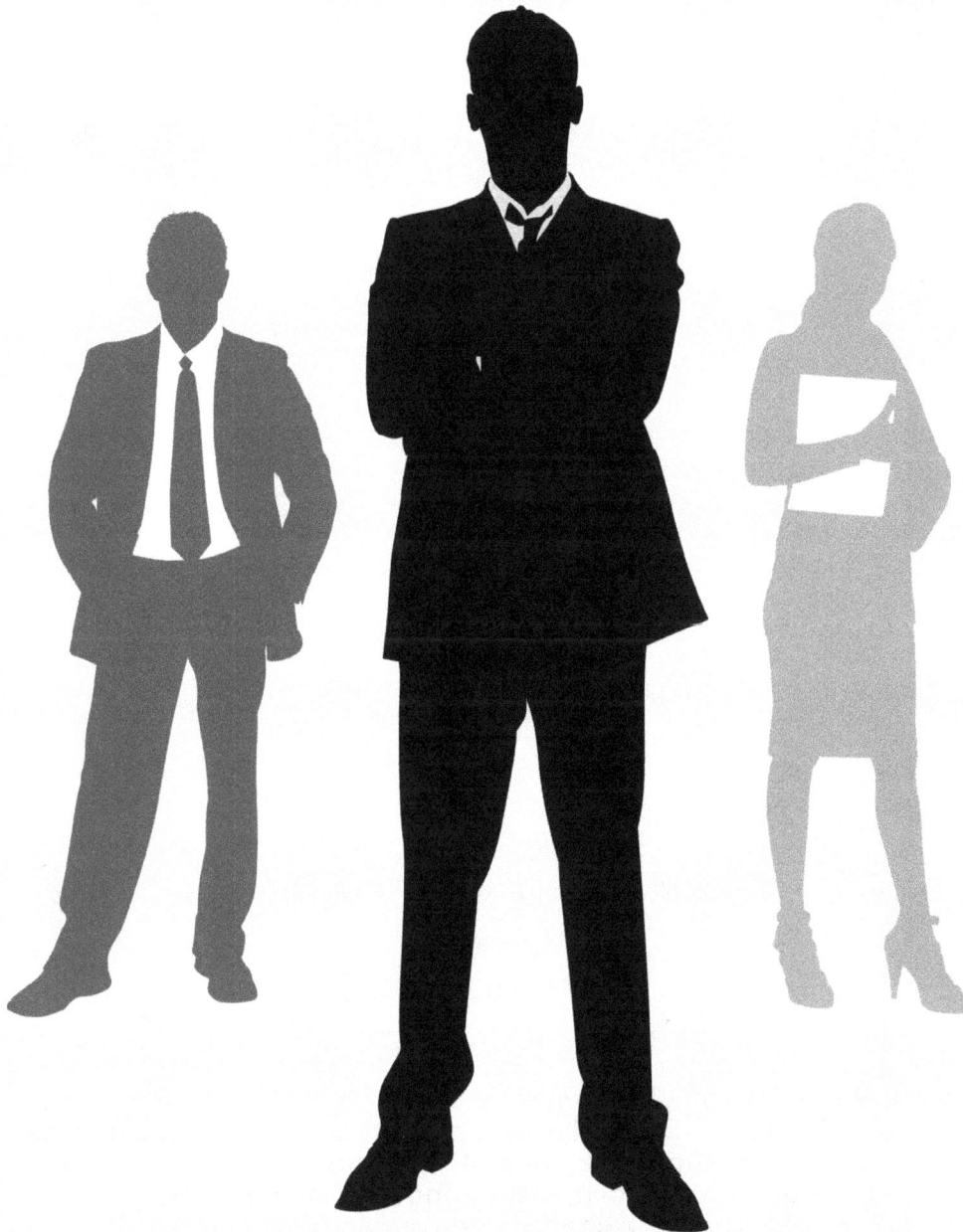

Michael P. O'Donnell, MBA, MPH, PhD
Alyssa Schultz, PhD

This workbook is published by the American Journal of Health Promotion. P.O. Box 1254, Troy, Michigan 48099-1254. Some of the contents are excerpted from Health Promotion in the Workplace, 4th Edition, to be published in 2014. For additional information about the 4th Edition e-mail contact@healthpromotionjournal.com.

The Employer's Business Case for Workplace Health Promotion

Michael P. O'Donnell, MBA, MPH, PhD
Alyssa Schultz, PhD

AMERICAN JOURNAL *of*

Health Promotion

Table of Contents

INTRODUCTION: WHY DO EMPLOYERS INVEST IN HEALTH PROMOTION PROGRAMS?

Approximately 94% of employers with 200 or more employees offer some form of **health promotion program**[1]. Furthermore, the percentage offering programs has been increasing[2,3] [See Tables 1 and 2]. This begs the question: "Why do employers invest in health promotion programs?" That is the focus of this chapter.

Table 1.

Percent of Employers Offering Health Promotion Programs at the Worksite according to Three Surveys[1,2,4]

Employer Size	2012	2010	2008
3-24	58%	74%	48%
25-199	79%	72%	69%
200-999	93%	91%	85%
1000-4999	96%	96%	91%
5000+	99%	98%	98%
All Employers	63%	74%	54%

Source: Kaiser Family Foundation and Health Research and Educational Trust. *Employer Health Benefits: 2012 Annual Survey.* Menlo Park, CA. 2012.

Employer Size	2011	2008	2005
<500	27%	19%	16%
500+	73%	57%	46%
10000+	77%	67%	47%
All Employers	44%	33%	27%

Source: MetLife. 10th Annual Study of Employee Benefits Trends. New York, NY, 2012.

Employer Size	1999	1992	1985
50-99	86%	75%	NA%
100-249	92%	86%	NA%
250-749	96%	90%	NA%
750+	98%	99%	NA%
All Employers	90%	80%	66%

Source: Association for Worksite Health Promotion, U.S. Department of Health and Human Services, William M. Mercer, Inc. *1999 National worksite health promotion survey.* Northbrook, IL: Association for Worksite Health Promotion and William M. Mercer, Inc. 2000.

* The 1985 survey did not measure program prevalence by employer size.

Table 2.

Percent of Employers Offering Specific Types of Health Promotion Programs at the Worksite

Type of Program	2004[5]	1999[2]	1992[6]	1985[6]
Blood pressure screenings	36%	29%	32%	NA*
Cholesterol screenings	29%	22%	20%	NA*
Cancer screening	22%	9%	12%	NA*
Health risk assessment	19%	18%	14%	NA*
Fitness programs	20%	25%	NA*	NA*
Nutrition or cholesterol education	23%	23%	NA*	NA*
Weight control classes or counseling	21%	14%	NA*	NA*
Quit smoking classes or counseling	19%	13%	NA*	NA*
Stress management classes or counseling	25%	26%	NA*	NA*
Alcohol or drug abuse programs	36%	28%	NA*	NA*

Back injury prevention	45%	53%	NA*	NA*
Maternal or prenatal programs	19%	12%	NA*	NA*
Balancing work/family education		18%	NA*	NA*
HIV/AIDS education	15%	25%	NA*	NA*
Workplace violence prevention programs		36%	NA*	NA*
Smoking policy	57%	79%	59%	27%

*Survey questions varied from year to year so not all categories are available for all years.

Historically, employers invested in health promotion programs to reduce medical care costs, improve productivity and enhance image[7,8]. Since most published research focuses on those areas, discussions of those studies will be the focus of this chapter. Savings in these areas can justify a health promotion program, just as savings in electricity can justify the cost of using a new energy efficient light bulb. However, a health promotion program that contributes only cost savings will suffer the same fate as a light bulb. When it burns out, it will be discarded.

A subtle but important shift in the way we perceive and investigate the financial—or broader organizational—return of a health promotion program may help to prevent such a fate. To survive and be successful, a health promotion program must contribute to the mission, long-term goals, and short-term priorities of the organization it serves and to the special interests of those who approve its budgets.

This concept was crystallized by the results of a benchmark study conducted more than a decade ago on the best health promotion programs in the United States[9]. This study illustrated that the best programs really did take a different approach to the direction and evaluation of their programs. Most of them have well-structured studies on health improvement, medical care cost savings, and **absenteeism** savings, but they also had something else. They had qualitative impressions of how their program contributed to the organization's mission, long-term goals, short-term goals, and the personal priorities of those who approved their funding. Studies that show medical care cost savings or absenteeism improvements are important only to the extent that controlling costs in these areas is an important priority for the organization. They might also be important if external visibility or **external validation** of their programs is one of the short- or long-term goals of the organization, or the priorities of the person approving the program.

An early survey of senior managers[2] lends further support for this conclusion. Only 4% of senior managers listed employee health as their top priority, and only 35% listed it as near the top of their priority list (see Table 3). Health promotion programs must be tied to the items that are near the top of the priority list for the entire organization to be perceived as important to the organization. Much of our future research and evaluation efforts must address this new area of concentration ... the impact of health promotion programs on the organization mission, long-term goals, short-term goals, and the personal priorities of those who approve their funding. It is important to recognize that different types of companies will have different reasons for implementing health promotion programs. For example, all industries, but particularly those with a high ratio of labor costs to total costs (such as hospitals or educational institutions), are concerned about health care costs and **productivity**. However, technology companies may be more focused on attracting and retaining top candidates for employment. Manufacturing industries may place top priority on avoiding employee injuries. Financial industries, whose employee demographics include a majority of younger females, may focus on work-life balance.

Table 3.

Where Does Employee Health and Well-Being Fall on Senior Management's Priority List? (Percentage of Companies)[2]

The number one priority	4%
Near the top of the priority list	35%
At the middle of the priority list	33%
Low on the priority list	16%
Not on the priority list	12%

The purpose of this chapter is to help readers understand why employers invest in health promotion programs. The conceptual argument and the evidence to date linking health promotion programs to medical care cost containment, productivity enhancement, and image enhancement are described. This is followed by a brief review of the methodological quality of the evidence. Side bar discussions recognize that the decision to start, continue, or discontinue a health promotion program are not always rational. Even so, employers can use this **conceptual framework** to project the financial impact of their program and to help them determine if a program will be a prudent investment for their organization.

Workplace Health Promotion in the United States and Around the World

This chapter primarily focuses on workplace health promotion in the United States where most large employers pay the health care costs of their employees. Under such a system, there is economic incentive for employers to become active in the area of employee health. In much of the rest of the world, employers do not pay those costs directly and so the reasons for investing in health promotion programs may be different than in the United States. A 1997 survey of European employers found the most important reasons for undertaking such programs were because of government legislation encouraging workplace health promotion, problems with employee morale, and productivity problems[10]. These reasons were cited by more than 60% of companies surveyed. When respondents were asked to report the associated benefits for the company, it was notable that significant benefits were perceived in the areas of staff morale, health problems, reduced turnover, and reduced accident rates[10].

A more recent study of European employers found a variety of **internal motivating factors** and **external motivating factors** for offering workplace health promotion[11]. Internal factors included evidence that programs had a significant impact on productivity, absenteeism, disability costs, job satisfaction, employee commitment, turnover, recruitment, and morale. Furthermore there was recognition that employee health and well-being are linked to accidents and injuries. Some of the external motivating factors reported by survey respondents were potential image enhancement for customers and future employees and support from local and government initiatives[11].

Apart from the specific goal of health care cost containment, many reasons for investing in workplace health promotion are similar for companies across the world. Improved employee health has the potential for impacting the organization in myriad positive ways. In the United States, the Patient Protection and Affordable Care Act of 2010 created new governmental incentives that encourage employers to offer workplace health promotion programs. Therefore, external motivating factors may provide additional incentives for employers to invest in such programs.

RATIONAL REASONS FOR INVESTING IN HEALTH PROMOTION PROGRAMS

There are a number of rational reasons employees invest in health promotion programs. The most widely cited among these are **medical care cost containment**, **productivity improvement**, and **image enhancement**.

Medical Care Cost Containment

Medical care costs have risen substantially during the past four decades in many developed nations around the world. Increases have been most dramatic in the United States. As a percent of gross domestic product (GDP), medical care costs in the United States have been increasing for 50 years, growing from 5.1% in 1960 to 7.1% in 1970, 9.0% in 1980, 12.4% in 1990, 13.7% in 2000, to 17.6% in 2010[12]. In dollars, medical care costs in the United States increased from $27.4 billion in 1960 to $2.6 trillion in 2010[13]. In 2010, the United States spent two and a half times as much on health care as the average of the 33 developed nations participating in the Organization for Economic Cooperation and Development at that time. On a per-capita basis, the United States spent an average of $8,233 per capita in 2010, which was 57% more than the Netherlands, the nation spending the second most.

These cost increases have been of special concern to employers because employers have assumed a disproportionate share of the increases. In 1965, employers paid 17% of the total cost, and employees paid 61%[14]. By 1989, employers paid 30%, and employees paid 37%, with the federal government covering the rest. By 1994, employers were paying 35.3%. As this trend has continued, employers have become much more aggressive about managing their costs and passing more costs on to employees; by 1999, employers were paying only 29.2% of total costs[15].

During the late 1980s and 1990s, employers implemented a wide range of medical care cost strategies, including sharing some costs with employees, training employees to be better consumers of medical care, forming coalitions of employers to negotiate bulk purchase discounts directly with medical care providers rather than insurers, and offering managed care as a preferred option—and sometimes the only option—to their employees. By 2000, an estimated 92,000,000 people were covered by **health maintenance organizations** (HMOs), compared to 54,000,000 in 1995 and 34,000,000 in 1990[16]. An estimated 92,000,000 additional people were members of preferred provider organizations (PPOs) by 1998[17]. Medical care providers also became very aggressive in their pricing. Development of health promotion programs was very compatible with these schemes and was often a part of cost-containment strategies. Although total medical care expenditures for the United States continued to increase in absolute dollars, as a percentage of GDP, medical care costs peaked in 1993 at 13.7%, dropped to 13.6% in 1994, increased to 13.7% in 1995, then dropped to 13.6% in 1996, and 13.4% in 1997[18]. Average medical care costs paid by employers seemed to be under control in the mid-1990s, dropping 1.1% in 1994, increasing only 0.2% in 1995, 1.4% in 1996, and dropping 2.9% in 1997[19].

Unfortunately, the success in medical care cost containment of the 1990s appeared to be short-lived, and in the early 2000s the **consumer-directed health plan** (CDHP), also known as **high-deductible health plans** became popular with employers in another effort to moderate costs. The creation of CDHPs stemmed from the assumption that a major driver of increased health care costs was that the patient (the consumer of health care) was insulated from the cost of care[20]. These plans combine a high-deductible health plan structure with health savings accounts or health reimbursement arrangements to promote cost-aware patient decision making. As of 2010, an estimated 12.6% of employees with employer-provided health coverage were enrolled in CDHPs[21], a rapid rise from just 4% in 2006[1].

The current spending on health care in the United States, 2.6 trillion dollars in 2010[13], is an incredible sum of money, and it is prudent business practice to take aggressive efforts to control it. A modest investment in health promotion that has a good chance of keeping employees healthy and out of the hospital is conceptually appealing, even without a lot of data to support the connection between health status and medical care costs, and most executives relied on their gut instincts to make decisions to invest in programs. However, in the past two decades, an impressive body of research has emerged to support this connection.

Health Risks are Associated with Medical Costs

The first significant study was conducted by Control Data Corporation[22]. After following 10,000 employees for four years, Control Data found that medical care claims were lowest for employees who exercised regularly, ate nutritious foods, fastened their seat belts, did not smoke cigarettes, and were not hypertensive. Similar results were found at Steelcase Corporation, an office furniture manufacturer[23,24]. Between 1985 and 1990, employees with zero risk factors had average annual medical care costs of only $250, while employees with six risk factors had costs of $1,600.

One of the early landmark studies[25] of the link between medical care costs and risk factors was produced through a collaboration of six employers (Chevron, Health Trust, Hoffman-La Roche, Marriott, State of Michigan, State of Tennessee) that was organized by the Health Enhancement Research Organization (HERO). StayWell (a health promotion vender) had health risk data and MEDSTAT (a medical care cost data management organization) had medical care cost data on these six employers. With the assistance of HERO and the permission of the employers, these two databases were merged to determine the relationship between ten **modifiable risk factors** and medical care costs. The strengths of this study include the large sample size, measurement of a wide range of risk factors, and the multivariate nature of the analysis. That study found eight risk factors (depression, stress, blood glucose, body weight, current or previous tobacco use, hypertension, and sedentary lifestyle) were associated with higher costs even after controlling for the other risk factors. That study was repeated again in 2012 with similar results. In that analysis, the health risks and costs of 92,486 people from seven companies were analyzed (see Table 4). Results again found that depression, blood glucose, blood pressure, body weight, tobacco use, physical inactivity, and stress were associated with higher costs after adjusting for all other risks.

Table 4.

Medical Care Costs Associated with Risk Factors[26]

Risk Factor	Mean Cost With Risk Factor	Mean Cost Without Risk Factor	% Difference (unadjusted)	% Difference (adjusted)
Depression	$6207	$3902	59.1%	48.0%
Stress	$5024	$4444	13.0%	8.6%
Blood glucose	$6532	$3842	70.0%	31.8%
Body weight	$4956	$3498	41.7%	27.4%
Tobacco use	$4192	$3784	10.8%	16.3%
Blood pressure	$5264	$4132	27.4%	31.6%
Exercise	$4477	$3537	26.6%	15.3%
Cholesterol	$4780	$4688	2.0%	-2.5%
Alcohol use	$3857	$4015	-3.9%	-9.5%
Nutrition	$3245	$4226	-23.2%	-5.2%

*The adjusted differences are the differences between those with and without each risk factor which persisted after adjusting for all of the other risk factors in a multivariate analysis. Costs are adjusted to 2009 dollars.

Costs were higher for those with elevated cholesterol but not after adjusting for the other nine risk factors. The finding that higher levels of alcohol consumption are not related to higher costs is initially surprising but has been found in other studies; people who drink excessively often neglect their health and do not seek medical care when they need it. The finding related to nutrition was surprising but also has been seen in other studies. This study showed the medical costs for those with good nutrition habits were actually higher both before and after adjustment. Our suspicion is that the tool used to measure nutrition habits within the questionnaire was too short to capture the full scope of nutrition habits that would impact health and medical care utilization. It was remarkable that the two studies published more than a decade apart had such consistent findings which lends credibility to the relationships found.

The 1998 HERO study also showed that employees who had a cluster of risk factors had strikingly higher costs. Employees with a cluster of seven heart disease risk factors had an average annual cost of $3,804, those with a cluster of risk factors for stroke had average annual cost of $2,349, and those with a cluster of psychological risk factors had average annual cost of $3,368. Employees with no risk factors had average costs of $1,166 (see Table 5). Others have found comparable results when examining different clusters of risk factors and points to the importance of addressing the whole person rather than just one risk factor at a time[27,28,29].

Table 5.

Medical Care Costs Associated with Clusters of Risk Factors, United States[25]

Risk Factor Cluster	With Risk Factors	Without Risk Factors	% Difference
Heart disease risks	$3,804	$1,158	228%
Stroke risks	$2,349	$1,272	85%
Psychosocial risks	$3,368	$1,368	147%
No risk factors		$1,166	

A related study coordinated by HERO[30], used the data from the 1998 investigation to estimate the percent of total costs attributable to these risk factors. The first study identified the most expensive risk factors among those who had these risk factors. The second study identified the total cost of the risk factors, factoring in the number of employees who had each of those risk factors. This changed the order of the most costly risk factors. For example, in the first study, depression was the most costly risk factor per person, but because less than 3% of employees in their sample suffered from depression, it did not have as significant an impact on total costs. Stress was the most costly risk factor because almost 20% of employees experienced high levels of stress. Almost 8% of total medical care costs were attributable to stress. Furthermore, this study showed that 24.9% of total costs were attributable to these 10 risk factors, all of which can be considered manageable through health promotion programs. This landmark study is very important because it indicates that 25% of annual medical care costs, or about $1,000 per employee, are attributable to risk factors that health promotion programs have been shown capable of managing. This information will better help an employer make a decision to invest the $50, $100, or $200 needed to pay for a program or at least will give the employer the objective data required to justify an emotional or gut level decision to invest in a program (see Table 6).

Table 6.

Cost of Risk Factors as a Percent of Total Medical Care Costs[30]

Risk Category	Cost/ High Risk	#At High Risk	Total Cost Due to Risk	% of Total Costs	Cost/ Capita
Stress	$732	8,518	$6,236,880	7.9%	$136
Former tobacco smoker	$311	14,329	$4,455,029	5.6%	$97
Body weight	$352	9,197	$3,239,919	4.1%	$70
Exercise habits	$173	14,908	$2,574,760	3.3%	$56
Current tobacco user	$228	8,797	$2,004,045	2.5%	$44
Blood glucose	$587	2,271	$1,332,646	1.7%	$29
Depression	$1,187	997	$1,183,439	1.5%	$26
Blood pressure	$199	1,827	$363,317	0.5%	$8
Excess alcohol use	-$52	1,723	-$89,027	-1.1%	$2
High cholesterol	-$14	8,641	-$117,431	-1.5%	-$3
Nutrition habits	-$162	9,278	-$1,500,623	-1.9%	-$33
Total expenditures attributable to high risk per capita			$19,682,953	24.9%	$428
Total medical care expenditures			$78,959,286		

A similar study was completed in South Korea and found analogous results[31]. Data on a randomly selected sample of over 180,000 employees were analyzed using a protocol similar to the HERO studies. This study found that employees with six heart disease risk factors had medical care costs 149% higher than those with none of these risk factors, and employees with three stroke risk factors had costs 52% higher than those with none of these risk factors (see Table 7). It is remarkable that similar trends persisted, even in a country where annual medical care costs are only one-eighth, or about $587 per year (1997 data), of those in the United States at that time[32].

Table 7.

Medical Care Costs Associated with Clusters of Risk Factors, South Korea[31]

Risk Factor Cluster	With Risk Factors	Without Risk Factors	% Difference
Heart disease risks	190,568 won	99,457 won	149%
Stroke risks	157,922 won	98,707 won	52%
No risk factors		41,515 won	

The work of the University of Michigan Health Management Research Center (UM-HMRC) provides additional support for the connection between health risks and medical costs. This Center has collected health care utilization and lifestyle behavior data during the past 30 years on more than 2,000,000 individuals working in more than 1,000 worksites. They have established long-term data management relationships with dozens of large employers. These data have allowed them to formulate and test a wide range of relationships between health risks and medical care costs, which are summarized in Table 8[33]. A number of these learnings are discussed in more detail.

Table 8.

Key Research Learning and Date Discovered, University of Michigan Health Management Research Center[33]

Learnings	Year Discovered

1. High-risk persons are high cost (prospective data)
   a. individual risks
   b. cumulative risks
	1991

2. Absenteeism and disability show the same relationship as medical costs	1993
3. Excess costs are related to excess risks	1993
4. Changes in costs (medical and pharmacy) follow changes in risks	1994
5. Risk combinations are the most dangerous predictors of cost	1995

6. Low-risk maintenance is an important program strategy	1996
7. Resource optimization: changes in risk drive changes in cost when targeted to specific risk combinations	1996
8. Wellness scores are highly correlated with medical costs	1997
9. Program participation is related to risk and cost moderation	1998
10. Wellness program opportunities are in preventive services, low- and high-risk interventions, and disease management	1998
11. Presenteeism is a measure of productivity and is associated with risks and disease	1999
12. Total value of health defined for the organization	2000
13. Natural flow of risks and costs; clusters of risks identified	2001
14. Focus on the person, not the risk or disease	2002
15. Time away from work responds to risks the same as medical costs	2002
16. Improved population health status as a result of employer-sponsored programs	2003
17. Benchmarks for bending population cost trend lines: 85%+ participation and 75%+ low-risks status	2004
18. Pre-retirement participation influences post-retirement participation	2005
19. Presenteeism changes follow risk changes	2005
20. "Don't get worse" philosophy, keep healthy people healthy	2006
21. Importance of culture of health	2007

After completing the UM-HMRCs **Health Risk Appraisal** (HRA), participants receive a personalized profile of their health risks as well as an overall score called a **wellness score**. The wellness score was found to be highly correlated with annual medical costs and is important because it allows a proxy measure of medical care costs that can be measured through a simple questionnaire.[34] These relationships are shown in Table 9.

Table 9.

Relationship between Wellness Score and Medical Care Costs[34]

Wellness Score	Annual Medical Costs
95	$1,415
90	$1,643
85	$1,800
80	$2,087
75	$2,369
70	$2,508
65	$2,817
60	$2,638
55	$2,818
50	$2,970

The relationship between medical care costs and health risks is further illustrated in Table 10, which shows the relative cost of high-risk versus low-risk conditions for actual illness, perceived health problems, physiological measures, and lifestyle habits. Not surprisingly, the difference in medical care costs is greatest for people who actually have a disease compared to those who do not have a disease, averaging 168% higher. Those who have risk factors measured by **biometric tests** have differences averaging 53% higher, which is very close to the differences for people who perceive problems related to health, satisfaction, and stress (48%). Costs for people with lifestyle risk factors are lowest among these four major categories but still average 16% higher than those without these risk factors.

Table 10.

Medical Care Costs and Health Factors[35]

Health Measure	Low Health Risk	High Health Risk	Difference
No Illness	$1773	$4168	140%
Disease			
Heart Disease	$1875	$8299	340%
Diabetes	$1975	$4669	140%
Cancer	$1981	$3456	70%
Other diseases	$1871	$4162	120%
raw average difference			168%
Biometric			
Blood pressure	$1810	$3732	110%
Relative body weight	$1881	$2633	40%
Cholesterol	$2033	$2276	10%
raw average difference			53%
Psychological Perceptions			
Physical health	$1751	$3756	110%
Life satisfaction	$2023	$2769	40%
Stress	$1857	$2572	30%

Job satisfaction	$2056	$2298	10%
raw average difference			48%
Lifestyle Habits			
Medication/ drug usage	$1874	$3034	60%
Physical activity	$1865	$2462	30%
Smoking	$2023	$2290	10%
Seat belt usage	$2059	$2007	-3%
Alcohol usage	$2072	$1695	-18%
raw average difference			16%

Health Risks are Associated with Other Cost Measures

In addition to medical costs, employee health risks have also been found to be associated with other health cost outcomes such as workers' compensation and pharmacy costs. In the 1980s and 1990s, pharmacy costs were a relatively minor component of employee health costs but they became the fastest rising contributor to total corporate health care costs[36] and represent the third-largest component of direct health care expenses after hospital care and physician services[37], comprising 15% of total health care spending in the United States[38]. As with medical claims, pharmacy claims have been found to be associated with employee health risks at corporations as diverse as a utility company[39] and a financial services organization[40]. The utility company found that approximately one-third of its pharmacy costs were attributed to excess health risks among the employees[39]. The financial services employer found that pharmacy costs increased in a stepwise manner as the number of employee health risks increased from zero to six or more[40].

Changes in Risks are Associated with Changes in Costs

After consistently finding that health risks measured by self-report questionnaire are associated with health care costs, the next logical question for the field was whether or not changes in those risks were associated with commensurate changes in health care costs. The UM-HMRC has published those results from several different organizations[41,42,43]. In 2001, Edington summarized the UM-HMRC's research based on their health risk and cost database containing more than 2,000,000 covered lives and with multiple years of data[44]. They found that health care costs decreased an average (median) of $153 with every one decrease in number of risk factors and increased an average (median) of $350 with every one increase in number of risk factors.

A more recent study[45] found similar results after examining pre- and post-HRA questionnaires taken by employees of six large employers. Medical and pharmaceutical claims were collected as the **outcome measure** for the duration of the study from 2004 to 2009. After controlling for chronic conditions, health risk changes from pre- to post-test were associated with health care cost changes in the year following the post-test. Employees with chronic conditions had a $129 reduction in cost for each risk reduced and an increase of $210 for each risk added while the costs of employees with no chronic conditions increased $101 for each risk added and decreased $25 for each risk reduced.

The finding that reduced risk factors are associated with reduced costs provides further support for the risk reduction programs advocated throughout this book. The finding that increases in risk factors are associated with increases in costs was a breakthrough discovery that led to the notion that keeping employees healthy was a worthy goal of health promotion programs in addition to reducing health risks among those with high risk factors. This is a critical finding because health promotion programs in the early days of our field were often criticized for attracting the people who already practiced healthy lifestyles. Programs do need to learn how to better attract those with unhealthy lifestyle practices, but the studies cited above underscore the importance of also helping those with healthy practices to continue those healthy practices.

Health Promotion Programs are Associated with Improvements in Risks and Costs

The link between medical costs and risk factors that can be modified by health promotion programs is fairly clear from the studies cited above. However, a separate question is whether health promotion programs can be successful in reducing employee health risks and ultimately in reducing health care costs. Dozens of studies have addressed this question, and a number of reviews have attempted to summarize the findings[46,47,48,49,50,51,52,53]. A large body of research has been compiled on the success of workplace health promotion programs in improving employee health risks, at least over the short-term. In terms of program impacts on costs, several literature reviews have attempted to summarize those findings. One such review was written by Aldana (1998)[54], who identified research on the impact of workplace health promotion programs on medical care costs. He then examined the methodology of each study, and determined which ones had **experimental**, **quasi-experimental** and **pre-experimental designs**. Aldana analyzed 24 studies: 21 (88%) of these studies showed that programs reduced medical care costs, and 3 (12%) showed no impact on medical care costs. Eight of the studies reported the cost of the program and the amount of savings achieved, thus allowing a calculation of the **cost/benefit ratio**. Savings ranged from $2.30 to $5.90 for every dollar invested and averaged $3.35. Also, the studies having experimental designs reported the highest levels of savings. Aldana repeated his analysis in 2001[55], with additional focus on assessing the quality of the research methodology. He reviewed 34 studies that examined the link between health risks (either single or multiple) and financial outcomes, 14 of which addressed health care costs, and 20 studies of absenteeism. The seven studies which presented **returns on investment (ROIs)** for health care cost savings found an average savings of $3.48 for every dollar spent on the program while three studies of absenteeism had an average ROI of 5.82. The majority of those reviewed studies received a "B" rating for the methodological quality (see Table 11).

Table 11.

Relationship between Health Risks and Health Care Costs and Absenteeism[61]

Health Risk	Number of Studies	Positive Relationship	Negative Relationship	No Relationship	Literature Rating	Conclusion
		Relationship between Health Risks and Health Care Costs				
Obesity	6	5	-	1	Indicative	Likely
Cholesterol	6	1	2	3	Weak	Inconclusive
Hypertension	5	4	-	1	Weak	Inconclusive
Stress	5	5	-	-	Indicative	Likely
Diet	2	-	2	-	Weak	Inconclusive

Alcohol Abuse	4	2	2	-	Weak	Inconclusive
Seat belt usage	2	1	-	1	Weak	Inconclusive
Fitness/ physical activity	6	3	-	3	Suggestive	Inconclusive
Multiple risk factors	5	5	-	-	Indicative	Likely
		Relationship between Health Risks and Absenteeism				
Obesity	5	5	1*	-	Indicative	Likely
Cholesterol	2	1	1	1[†]	Weak	Inconclusive
Stress	8	7	-	1	Indicative	Likely
Fitness/ physical activity	7	2	-	5	Weak	Inconclusive
Hypertension	5	2	-	3	Weak	Inconclusive
Multiple risk factors	3	3	-	-	Indicative	Likely
Diet	0	-	-	-	No data	No data
Alcohol abuse	0	-	-	-	No data	No data
Seat belt use	0	-	-	-	No data	No data

* All five studies found that more obese women had higher absenteeism levels; four studies found that more obese men had higher absenteeism levels; one found that more obese men had lower absenteeism levels.

[†] One study found that employees with high cholesterol had higher rates of absenteeism; the other found that women with high cholesterol had lower rates of absenteeism, but there was no relationship for men.

Chapman conducted a meta-analysis of ROI studies in 2003, 2005 and again in 2012 with somewhat more lenient inclusion criteria[56,57,58]. By 2012, his review included a total of 62 studies about the economic return of worksite health promotion programs. The methodological quality scores for those 62 studies ranged from 12 to 30 points, reflecting a wide variation in quality of research in our field although the more recent studies had larger sample sizes and higher quality methods and received more weighting in the meta-analysis. The final result of the meta-evaluation found an average cost/benefit ratio of 5.56 across 25 studies which reported a cost/benefit ratio including benefits from health costs, sickness absenteeism, workers' compensation and disease management costs.

In the same year, Baicker and colleagues completed a meta-analysis of the literature on health costs and savings associated with workplace health promotion programs[59]. **Meta-analysis** is a method of systematically combining data from similar studies and repeating the analysis with the combined larger data set. It often allows trends to be identified that were not apparent in the individual studies. Baicker's analysis included 22 studies, primarily conducted at large employers, and found that medical costs decreased $3.27 for every dollar spent on employee wellness programs. It is important to note that nearly all ROI analyses of workplace wellness programs have been limited to programs offered by large employers. Smaller employers may be less likely to have the **economies of scale** required to demonstrate a return on investment from health promotion programs but it does not mean that they would not receive benefits from such programs.

How should we interpret the above findings? It is likely that studies that found negative or neutral results were not submitted for publication or were more likely to be rejected if they were submitted. Nevertheless, the trend of positive ROIs is very encouraging. We can conservatively conclude based on the research that some health promotion programs are clearly able to reduce medical care costs. We can also conclude that some programs are apparently able to produce medical care cost savings that far exceed their cost. We need to put these cost/benefit values in perspective. An employer never expects to make money on an employee benefit (like a health promotion program) and rarely, if ever, expects the program to pay for itself in directly measurable savings. Almost any employer would be more than satisfied with an employee benefit that produces a cost/benefit ratio of 1.00 which means $1.00 in savings for every $1.00 invested; returns of $3.00 for every dollar invested are clearly outstanding.

In conclusion, the relationship between medical care costs and risk factors that can be modified by health promotion programs is strong. Also, research on the impact of programs on medical care costs does support the claim that programs can reduce medical care costs. The quality of the research methodology is also adequate. This body of research should be sufficient to persuade an employer that health promotion programs can moderate medical costs. We could not make this statement in the early years of this field. Furthermore, we can probably increase the savings potential of health promotion programs if we design programs with the explicit goal of impacting medical care costs. To do this, we need to focus more attention on the health risks that are most costly, such as injury and musculoskelatal problems, instead of the health risks with the strongest links to death and chronic disease, such as cardiovascular disease and cancer. At the same time we need to address the needs of low-risk employees by providing them with encouragement and opportunities to remain healthy and stay low-risk. Many programs have already adopted the strategy of focusing on high-risk employees, but few have recognized the importance of keeping healthy employees healthy as a strategic focus[60]. We also need to incorporate programs on the wise use of medical services and encourage appropriate use of pharmaceuticals and medical care, particularly for those with chronic health conditions such as diabetes or asthma. A large percentage of services provided are medically unnecessary, and it is possible to educate employees to use care more appropriately.

Productivity Enhancement

We have long argued that health promotion programs enhance productivity, and as the research improves, we have more and more evidence to support this claim. Historically, research focused on employee absenteeism[24,61,62], then additional measures of workers' compensation absences[63], and short- and long-term disability outcomes were studied[64,65]. Finally, measures of on-the-job productivity losses, also known as **presenteeism**, were included in health promotion research. Productivity at work is difficult to measure, particularly in knowledge-based jobs. In general terms, employee productivity is defined as output per unit of labor. Among blue-collar workers, this might be measured in terms of automobiles, toys, tables, or any other product produced per hour. For white-collar workers, it might be designs created, insurance claims processed, or customer service calls handled per hour. For a sales person, it might be sales closed per month, and for a film producer, it might be films produced per year. In addition to the quantity of units produced, the quality of each unit produced is an important element of productivity; the automobiles, toys, and tables must meet all production standards. To be of value to the organization, designs, claims processed, and service calls taken must be free of errors. The sales closed must not be canceled, and the films made must be well made.

Within the health promotion community, most of the focus to date on productivity has been on absenteeism, primarily because absenteeism is easy to measure, but also because absenteeism is an important part of productivity. When a worker is absent, s/he may continue to get paid but produces no work. In some cases, s/he is replaced by someone else who must be paid. This raises the cost of producing the same level of output. In other cases, he or she is not replaced, and co-workers are required to disrupt their work to fill in for the absent employee. This reduces total output. In either case, output per unit of labor (i.e., productivity) drops. Health promotion programs are expected to reduce absenteeism by helping people stay healthy and thus reduce the need to be absent. This is reasonable as long as illness is the cause of the absence. Sometimes people take a "mental health" day when they need a break. Other times they call in sick when, in fact, they are staying home with a sick child. The impact of a health promotion program on these cases is more complex and is better explained within a broader conceptual approach, which is illustrated in Figure 1.

Figure 1.

Mechanisms linking health, productivity and profit.[91]

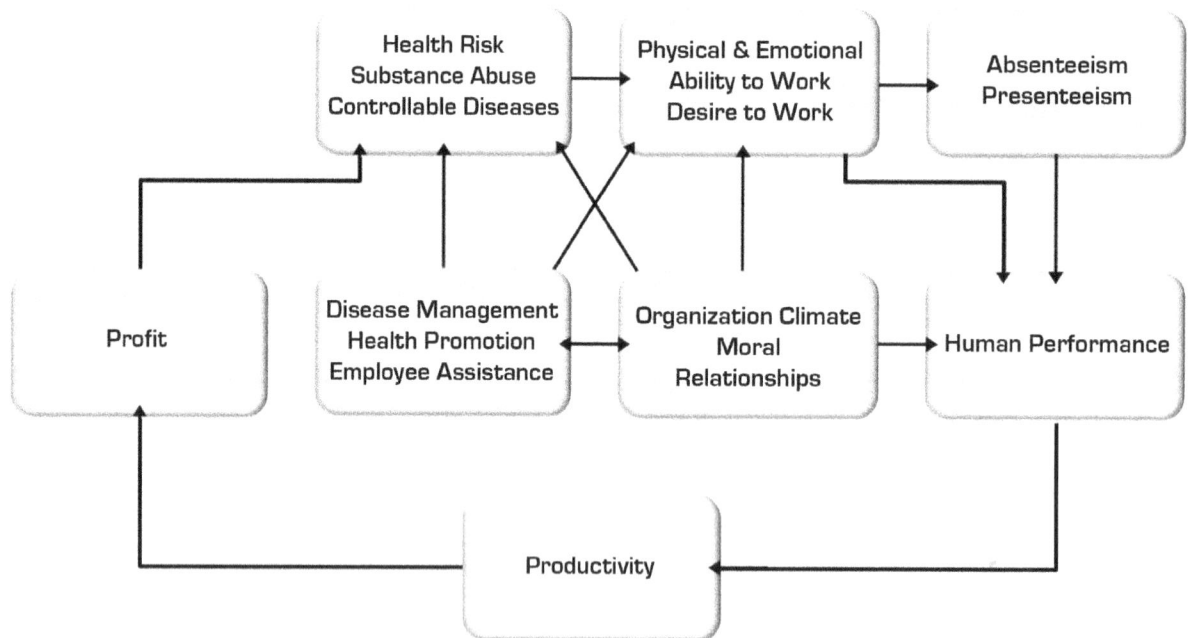

The Concept

The basic concept, as illustrated in Figure 1, is that human performance is higher when people are physically and emotionally able to work and have the desire to work. Higher levels of human performance lead to higher levels of productivity, which in turn can lead to higher profit levels. Health promotion programs play a central role in this model because they can improve health by reducing health risks, helping to manage controllable diseases, and reducing use of mood-altering substances. These health improvements lead to improved physical and emotional ability to work. Health promotion programs also improve **organization climate**, which enhances people's desire to work and directly enhances human performance. This model also asserts that improved organization climate and higher profit levels directly reduce health risks. This is a preliminary model that must be tested and refined. Elements within the model may change and new mechanisms may be discovered.

Why Is This Concept of Enhancing Productivity So Important?

The basic reason is that increased human productivity can lead to increased profits. In operational terms, higher productivity in a manufacturing setting means more product is produced with fewer labor hours of input. Increased productivity in research and development means more and better product enhancements emerge from research labs. Increased productivity in sales and marketing means more products are sold and sales revenues are higher. Increased productivity in management means people receive more effective guidance and coordination. Productivity enhancement has always been important for these reasons, but is even more important as businesses compete globally.

Corporations' desire to improve productivity is also important because American businesses have entered an increasingly competitive global business environment. American businesses lead the world in most measures of productivity[66]; however, labor costs in the United States are among the highest in the world, and U.S. markets have fewer limitations on imports than virtually any other major market in the world. If U.S. businesses want to continue to compete successfully, they must have higher quality products produced at lower cost through more productive processes. Finally, existing developments in computer technology and emerging developments in **measurement theory** are enabling businesses to measure productivity with greater accuracy and efficiency than ever before. Just as double digit medical care cost increases in the 1970s sparked a decades-long focus on medical care cost containment, this combination of events has sparked what we expect will be a decades-long focus on productivity enhancement.

How much more productive will employees be who are physically and emotionally able to work and motivated to work because they feel their employer is concerned about their well-being? This remains an open question; one that we expect will receive considerable attention in the next decade. The author has posed this question in formal discussions with hundreds of executives and dozens of scientists during the past few decades. The most common response from scientists is that employees will be 5% to 10% more productive. The most common response from executives is that employees will be 100% more productive! As we would expect and hope, scientists are more conservative in their estimates. However, executives think of themselves when they answer this question. They know how much more productive they are when they are full of energy, not distracted by emotional problems, and really want to work. They know they are far more likely to be effective in their creative thinking, negotiating, efforts to motivate people, strategic planning, and any other challenging activity when they feel good and are motivated. In reality, a factory worker or clerk who has little control over his or her work environment might be able to increase productivity by 5%, 10%, or even 30%. A knowledge worker, such as a lawyer, scientist, writer, salesperson, or senior manager, might be able to increase productivity by 50%, 100%, or even more.

To make this relevant to business, we need to quantify the value of productivity increases and losses. The data supporting a financial payoff from health promotion are probably strongest in the area of medical cost savings, but the greatest potential payoff for health promotion is probably in productivity enhancement. The reason for this is simple. The maximum benefit we can achieve in medical cost savings is to eliminate the cost, or more realistically, to eliminate the costs related to lifestyle risk factors. If we eliminate the total medical care cost, this will save approximately $6,000 per year per covered life (employee + dependents). If we eliminate the 25% of costs that are related to lifestyle risk factors, we will save approximately $1,500 per year per employee. More realistically, if we eliminate one quarter of the 25% of costs that are related to lifestyle risk factors, we will save approximately $375 per year per employee. Savings at any of these levels would be significant and more than enough to pay for the health promotion program, but they are minor compared to the additional revenue and profit we could earn by increasing productivity.

If productivity increases by 1% in a company with a 10% profit margin and that increased productivity can be translated into increased revenues, this will increase profits by 10%. If the profit margin is 5%, profits will increase by 20%. If productivity increases by 10%, profits will increase by 100% with a 10% profit margin and by 200% with a 5% profit margin. A 1% increase in profits in the United States in 2012[67] would be worth $150 billion per year, a 10% increase worth $1.5 trillion, and a 20% increase worth $3.0 trillion. Potential returns of this magnitude will grab the attention of even the most skeptical executives and policy makers.

Measuring productivity is very difficult and measuring the on-the-job productivity losses associated with poor health (presenteeism) has been a topic of great interest in recent years. Dozens of **presenteeism questionnaires** have been created and tested in a variety of settings. Several reviews of these instruments and their use in employee populations have been published[68,69,70,71]. In general, these productivity loss instruments have been found to be **valid** and **reliable** in measuring the association between health conditions and health risks with on-the-job productivity in a variety of jobs and industries. In one study, an objective measure of productivity was used with telephone customer service operators in order to assess the relationship between health risks (measured by an HRA) and productivity at work[72]. As the number of health risks increased, employee productivity decreased; and disease states were associated with productivity reduction as well. Measuring productivity among telephone operators who are "plugged in" during their entire shift is not easily replicated in most other occupations. Hence, the presenteeism questionnaires attempt to quantify the loss of productivity in several different ways such as the physical demands of work, interpersonal communication, getting to work on time, working a full shift, and quality of work accomplished.

While it appears that we can reliably state that health risks and health conditions are associated with a certain degree of productivity loss on the job, there is much less agreement on whether or not we can monetize those results[73,74]. Presenteeism instruments have given wildly varying estimates of the cost of presenteeism associated with several health risks and conditions. But it is unknown exactly how those productivity estimates can be translated into dollars for the organization. If a worker is 10% less productive today because she is suffering from a migraine, does she work twice as hard to-morrow to catch up the work she couldn't get to the day before? Or, if a database programmer needs to take a stretch break every 20 minutes to alleviate back pain, is that time lost or is it recouped when the worker returns to his desk with renewed energy? How do you accurately measure the productivity of a knowledge based worker who may arrive at a solution to a design flaw while he or she is not even at work? In many situations, workers put in extra hours to make up for lost time on a previous day, or co-workers shoulder a heavier load while co-workers are not well. All of these factors create a very complex context in which to calculate the dollar losses associated with presenteeism.

Measuring the impact of health promotion programs on productivity is even more difficult. As we recognized above, most early efforts to measure the impact of health promotion on productivity have focused on absenteeism as an outcome measure. Aldana[54] reviewed the research on the impact of absenteeism on productivity. He found 16 studies on this topic; 14 (87%) of the studies reported reductions in absenteeism after the introduction of the health promotion programs, one study reported no change, and one study reported an increase in absenteeism as a result of the program. Five of the studies reported cost/benefit analysis values, with a range of $2.50 to $10.10 saved for every $1.00 invested and an average savings of $4.90. The studies with experimental designs had the highest level of savings values (see Table 11).

In 2004, a study of 500 employees found that a reduction of one health risk improved presenteeism by 9% after controlling for baseline risks and demographic factors[75]. A similar study[76] measured changes in presenteeism using a modified version of the Work Limitations Questionnaire and compared it with changes in health risks over a two-year period. Each risk factor increased or reduced from 2002 to 2004 was associated with a commensurate change of 1.9% productivity loss. Mills and colleagues[77] conducted a quasi-experimental study to evaluate the impact of a comprehensive health promotion program on employee health risks and work productivity measured by the Work Performance Questionnaire. They found that the intervention group of employees had a significant improvement in work performance compared to the control group after twelve months of follow-up.

One study combined the outcome measures of absenteeism, short-term disability, and workers' compensation into a sum of the cost of **time away from work (TAW)** and compared it with health risk status and individual health risks of 6,220 hourly workers at Steelcase Inc. from 1998 to 2000[64]. Higher TAW costs were associated with several individual health risks and Table 12 shows the association of overall health risk status with TAW which helps to illustrate the total value of employee health to the organization. The excess costs associated with excess health risks accounted for 36% of the costs totaled for medical, pharmacy, absence, disability and workers' compensation at the study corporation[64]. The importance of this concept is that much of what individuals and companies spend on health is excess relative to a baseline population of those with zero, one or two health risks (overall low-risk status).

Table 12.

Total Value of Health: Excess Costs associated with Excess Risks[64]

Outcome Measure	Low Risk	Medium Risk	High Risk	Excess Cost Percentage*
Short-term Disability	$120	$216	$333	41%
Workers' Compensation	$228	$244	$496	24%
Absence	$245	$341	$527	29%
Medical & Pharmacy	$1,158	$,1487	$,3696	38%
Total	$1,751	$2,288	$5,052	36%

*Excess cost column reflects the number of employees in each of the risk categories

Loeppke reviewed the research on the total value of health to individuals, corporations, populations and nations and concluded that there is good evidence that health promotion can lower health risks, reduce the burden of disease, improve productivity, and lower total health costs. He found the most important driving factors of successful programs to be the commitment to prevention and having the ultimate goal of creating a culture of health within organizations and communities[78]. It appears that business leaders agree. A recent survey of employers' health care strategies in 2012 by the Towers Watson/National Business Group on Health found that "developing a workplace culture where employees are accountable and supported for their health and well-being" was cited as a top focus area by 40% of respondents, the most frequently reported answer[79].

The above results are very encouraging, and we should be comfortable in concluding that some health promotion programs can reduce absenteeism and presenteeism and that, in some cases, the savings in absenteeism may more than pay for the cost of the program. However, we are not yet comfortable in quantifying the monetary savings in improvements in on-the-job productivity.

Image Enhancement

We have very little data to support the impact of health promotion on company image, and most of it is out of date, but it remains a very important motivation for many employers who develop health promotion programs. In an early survey, attracting new employees was identified as an important reason for developing a health promotion program by 67% of employers and retaining existing employees was cited by 76% of employers[2].

Some of the early health promotion programs were developed primarily for image-related reasons. For example, when the Silicon Valley was emerging in the 1970s, engineers were in great demand. Companies such as Apple, Advanced Micro Devices, and Hewlett-Packard were growing from zero to thousands of employees in just a few years. College graduates with bachelor's degrees were commanding salaries of $50,000, which is the equivalent of about $250,000 in 2012 dollars. Also, many of these companies were developing competitive products with great growth potential. Knowledge of how to develop these products had great market value, so retaining existing employees was even more important than attracting new ones.

Many of these companies realized they could not survive financially by competing for employees solely through salaries; it was much less expensive, and initially more distinctive and effective, to compete based on benefits. For example, an elaborate club-type fitness center could be built for an amortized cost of $500 per employee per year and serve as a beacon to new employees and a morale-boosting perk for existing employees. If that same $500 were added to an employee's salary, it would work out to an increase of about $0.24 an hour, even less after taxes. Most professional employees already earning a large salary would not even notice such an increase. The Silicon Valley is a unique environment, but we have seen similar growth of new health promotion programs in other geographic areas that have gone through rapid industrial growth.

Some companies add health promotion programs when it is consistent with their products. For example, during the late 1970s and early 1980s, over half of the hospitals in the United States started selling health promotion programs to corporations and individuals in their communities. Prospective employer clients naturally asked these hospitals how well the health promotion program for their own hospital employees was working. Most of these hospitals did not initially have programs in place but scrambled to launch them. Unfortunately, when hospitals realized it was very difficult to run a profitable hospital-based health promotion program, many discontinued their corporate and community programs, as well as their internal employee health promotion programs and most of these programs shut down. In recent years, there has been a growing interest in hospital health promotion, and the American Hospital Association is stepping up to provide guidance. This has manifested in their recently released report: A Call to Action, Creating a Culture of Health[80], which encourages hospitals to take a leadership role in developing health promotion in their communities, starting with developing excellent health promotion programs for their own employees.

Programs also seem to develop in industry clusters. For example, health promotion programs are common among employers in high technology, oil, insurance, consumer products, public utilities, government agencies, and, automotive companies. This industry **cluster effect** illustrates how benefits are typically added. A rational perspective would lead us to conclude that companies conduct organized prospective cost/benefit analyses to decide which benefits to add and retain. As discussed below, a rational analysis is not always the driving force in decisions about health promotion programs. How many companies have ever tried to measure the impact of their medical care coverage on productivity or even on the health of their employees? Very few. Instead, companies typically look at the benefits offered by their primary competitors and try to match those benefits. This does not mean that they spend their dollars frivolously. They are very aggressive in securing the best price/quality balance and in containing overall costs of their benefits... they just don't use the methods we might expect them to use to select benefits based on the returns they provide.

The auto industry in Detroit provides a good example of the clustering effect, the desire to have benefits comparable to competitors, and the nonscientific method by which programs are often added. In the Detroit area, large automobile companies set the standard of high pay and excellent benefits. This started when the first large auto company was started by Henry Ford. Much like the high technology companies in California in the 1970s (and the present day), Henry Ford needed to hire a huge number of employees to keep up with the exploding demand for cars created when he was able to reduce the cost of each car with the development of the assembly line. He offered hourly wages that were more than double the normal wages for a factory worker. Until recently, the labor unions have been successful in keeping those wages and benefits above market levels. Major employers in the Detroit area set their salary and benefit packages to try to keep up with the automobile companies. During the early 1980s, Ford, then Chrysler, started to add employee health promotion programs. These programs continued to grow in the late 1980s and 1990s despite the fact that in 1991 the United States auto industry had the worst financial performance in its history. Ford, Chrysler, and General Motors lost a combined $7.5 billion in 1991[81]. A few years later, General Motors began developing plans for its employee health promotion program, a program that was once the largest employee health promotion program in the United States and probably the world. General Motors did have good rational reasons to develop a program: they were the only major U.S. auto company that did not have a program, and they had a relatively old work force and very high medical care costs. Despite these rational motivators, the impetus came from two new members of their corporate board, one of whom was a previous Secretary of Health and Human Services. These board members figured out how to divert existing health-care-related funds; within a few months, efforts to develop a program were underway. Following the lead of the auto companies, employers in southeastern Michigan have continued to develop and maintain employee health promotion programs. By the early 2000s, health promotion had become part of the culture and business strategy for auto companies, which is probably the primary reason they maintained their programs even when several of them nearly went bankrupt in 2007.

This desire to match the benefits of major competitors is likely responsible for some of the spread of health promotion to workplaces internationally. As companies around the world compete globally, they need to establish an image at least as polished as their major American competitors. They also need to recruit employees from the same labor pools, and having comparable benefits will be part of the strategy to achieve this. This will be especially true in Asia, where establishing position and saving 'face' is such an important part of the culture.

Combined Motives

It is important to stress that most organizations will have multiple motives for establishing their health promotion programs; some of these motives may not be entirely rational (See side bar: A Counter Perspective: The Emotional Factor). Also, as suggested by Green and Cargo nearly two decades ago[82], health promotion programs are so common now that some employers will adopt programs because they realize health promotion makes good business sense. A process to help managers determine if a proposed health promotion program is likely to produce sufficient returns is described in the side bar titled "How Can an Employer Determine if a Health Promotion Program Will Be a Good Investment?"

Table 13.

Reasons Contributing to a
Business Decision to Offer Health Promotion Program[19]

Keep workers healthy	84%
Improve morale	77%
Retain good employees	76%
Reduce medical care costs	75%
Attract good employees	67%
Improve productivity	64%

How Good Is the Quality of the Evidence?

In 1984, we could only speculate about the financial impact of health promotion programs. Only a handful of studies had been published, and all of them had serious methodological flaws. By 1994, hundreds of studies had been published on the impact of

A COUNTER PERSPECTIVE: THE EMOTIONAL FACTOR

Why, indeed, do employers invest in health promotion programs for their employees? In the past four decades we have spent untold hours examining this question. We have felt our efforts to answer this question were well spent, because the future of our programs depended on this data. We were right in that feeling, but we may have made a basic mistake in our assumptions.

We have assumed that a decision to invest in a health promotion program is made through a fully rational process, and we have scrambled to accumulate data that show the financial returns of programs.

Ironically, now that we have good data to support the financial returns that can be realized from health promotion programs, we need to recognize that this process of deciding to start or continue a program is not fully rational.

Basically, what we need to start or continue a health promotion program is the emotional buy-in of the person who has the authority to say "YES," the emotional buy-in of the individual who has the authority to approve spending of $100 to $250 per employee per year. That's how much health promotion programs cost. To most organizations that is not very much. On the lower end, it is the equivalent of taking all the employees out for a holiday dinner. At the upper end, it is about as much as landscaping or carpeting a new facility. Spending at this level is not frivolous. Spending at this level does require close supervision to make sure the money is well-spent. However, it does not require the level of sophisticated cost/benefit analysis we have conducted to defend health promotion investments. Major investments, such as the acquisition of another company or the launch of a new product, often have less data to support their returns than we have to support investments in health promotion.

If a health promotion program has the emotional buy-in of top management, it will be approved and continued[33,83]. If not, the program will never start or will be discontinued when budget problems occur. In a small- to medium-sized company, the president will have sufficient authority to approve investment in a health promotion program. In a large company, a senior vice president will have authority to make an investment of this order of magnitude.

The authors have come to this conclusion based primarily on experience in talking to the top managers who have approved, continued, and discontinued programs. However, there are a few studies that support this position. For example, a study by Wolfe, Slack, and Rose-Hearn[84] of a small group of Canadian companies showed that senior managers did not list financial savings as the primary management motivation for establishing and continuing programs, although program managers did. Senior managers wanted to enhance morale, and they were not looking for direct quantifiable financial returns. At a personal level, Gerry Greenwald, former Chairman and Chief Executive Officer of United Airlines and former Chairman of Chrysler Motors asked one of the authors if there was any evidence to show that programs work, especially if they save money. After hearing the findings from a dozen studies, he stopped the presentation, saying that was more than enough to convince him and that he usually had far less evidence to guide him in making investment decisions of hundreds of millions of dollars.

From another perspective, some employers have a philosophical opposition to interfering with employees' private lives, health habits and medical decision-making[85] and will be unlikely to ever invest in health promotion at the workplace.

Also, an early national survey of employers conducted by William M. Mercer, Inc., for the Department of Health and Human Services[19], "keeping employees healthy" was cited by 84% of employers as an important reason for establishing a program. Reducing medical care costs was listed by 75%, and improving productivity was listed by 64% (see Table 13). Cost containment was important but not the most important reason.

The Dupont and Pacific Bell health promotion programs may provide further support for this concept. Both of these programs received the C. Everett Koop Award from the Health Project in encouraging researchers to conduct higher quality studies. Both had published good quality studies illustrating cost savings[86,87], yet both programs were discontinued. The reasons these programs were discontinued were never publicized, so we cannot conclude that an "emotional" factor was the cause. However, we can conclude that something other than the medical care cost containment or absenteeism reduction outcomes, which these programs demonstrated, was more important to their respective organizations.

The authors have always been, and continue to be, strong advocates for excellent program evaluation and research on the health and financial benefit of health promotion programs, but think it is important that we be more aware of why and how organizations make decisions to develop and continue or discontinue programs. To be successful and survive, a health promotion program must contribute to the mission, long-term goals, and short-term priorities of the organization it serves, and to the special interests of those who approve its budgets. Sometimes these specific interests are unstated emotional factors. Our research and evaluation efforts should address all of these factors.

workplace health promotion programs; a large number of them addressed financial outcomes. Our general conclusion at that time was that most of the studies did have some flaws in methodology that prevented us from making conclusive statements that programs do save money. We devoted a great deal of time examining the methodological flaws of the research and recognition of the outstanding quality of these programs. It is still important for practitioners to be aware of these problems, so we are including a list (see Table 14) on the most common potential threats to internal validity[88]. Despite these flaws, we made it very clear that the amount and quality of research supporting the financial returns from health promotion programs was, even then, far superior to the research supporting business investments for decisions with costs similar to those of a health promotion program. After all, these programs cost from only $50 (or less) per employee for a basic program to $350 for the best comprehensive programs in the country. As mentioned earlier, this cost is about as much as a year-end party, carpeting, landscaping, etc. The quality of the evidence we had in 1994 was more than sufficient for an employer to make a decision to invest in a health promotion program. Indeed, by 1990, 81% of employers surveyed had decided to develop some form of health promotion program[2]. Since 1994, numerous additional studies had been published, and the quality of studies continued to improve. By 2002, the outcomes in our field of research expanded to include multiple measures of productivity, and the number of employers who scientifically evaluated the success of their programs grew. We had examples of successful programs in many types of organizations with diverse workforces and from varying industries and geographic locations.

Table 14.

Potential Threats to Internal Validity[88]

Validity Threat	Definition/Description
1. Selection	A threat when effect may be due to pre-existing differences between the kinds of people in the study groups.
2. Attrition	Refers to the dropping out of subjects over time such that the characteristics of remaining subjects at posttest are different from the characteristics of the full group at pretest. In multiple group studies, differential mortality occurs when the characteristics of subjects leaving the study are different between the experimental and comparison groups.
3. Maturation	Processes occurring within the respondents as a function of the passage of time; growing older, more experienced, more motivated. In multiple group studies, selection may interact with maturation such that respondents in one group "mature" faster than respondents in another group, regardless of the treatment.
4. History	Refers to the specific unintended events occurring between the pretest and posttest measurements in addition to the treatment variable. In multiple group studies, local history is a threat when events other than the treatment affect one group but not another.
5. Instrumentation	Operates due to improper precalibration of measuring instrument: changes in the calibration of the instrument between the pretest and posttest; or because scale intervals are not equal and change is easier to detect at some points on the measurement scale than on others.
6. Statistical Regression	Tendency for an unusually high or low score to regress or return to a more usual or mean level on subsequent measures.
7. Treatment Fidelity	Refers to the ability to infer that the treatment, or worksite health promotion program, exists in sufficient strength to cause the intended outcome.
8. Diffusion of Treatments	Occurs when experimental and comparison groups have contact, and the comparison group may receive the treatment or part of the treatment from the experimental group.

9. Testing	The effects of taking a test upon the scores of a future testing. Also referred to as **reactiveness of measures.**
10. Compensatory Rivalry among Respondents Receiving the Less Desirable/No Treatment	May operate in multiple group studies when rivalry is engendered among the subject receiving the less desirable treatment or no treatment. Also referred to as the **John Henry effect.**
11. Resentful Demoralization of Respondents Receiving the Less Desirable/No Treatment	May operate in multiple group studies when the comparison group gets discouraged because they were not given the favorable treatment and, as a result, their behavior is negatively affected.
12. Compensatory Equalization of Treatments by Administrators	May operate in multiple group studies when there is administrative reluctance to tolerate inequality of treatments among groups.
13. Ambiguity about the Direction of Causal Influence	Not clear if A caused B or B caused A.

The Aldana reviews[54,55] and the Baicker et al. review[59] cited previously are probably the best reviews of the literature on the financial impact of workplace health promotion programs from the perspective of having a systematic search process, factoring in methodology quality and summarizing results of the literature as a whole. In addition to summarizing the impact of the studies, the Aldana review also critiqued the methodology of each study using the criteria in Table 15.

Table 15.

Definitions of the Various Scoring Criteria[61]

	Description
Study Rating	
A	Properly randomized, controlled study (experimental designs).
B	Well-designed controlled trials without randomization (quasi-experimental designs).
C	Well-designed cohort or case-control studies (pre-experimental designs).
D	Trend data, correlational and regression studies (correlational designs).
E	Expert opinions, descriptive studies, case reports, reports of expert committees.
Literature Rating	
Weak	Research evidence supporting relationship is fragmentary, nonexperimental, and/or poorly operationalized. A majority of experts in the field believe causal impact is plausible but no more so than alternative explanations.
Suggestive	Multiple studies consistent with relationship, but no randomized control groups. Most experts believe causal impact is consistent with knowledge in related areas but see support as limited and acknowledge plausible alternative explanations.
Indicative	Relationship supported by substantial number of well-designed studies, with few or no randomized control groups. Experts believe that relationship is likely causal, but evidence is still tentative.
Acceptable	Cause-effect relationship supported by well-designed studies with randomized control groups.
Conclusive	Cause-effect relationship between intervention and outcome; substantial number of well-designed, randomized, control studies.

The most important methodological problems in the research on the financial impact of workplace health promotion programs have not changed much in the past decade; they include lack of sufficient randomized controlled designs, small sample sizes, short duration of the studies, inadequate measurement tools, and inappropriate analysis[54]. Despite these limitations, it is difficult to find many higher quality bodies of research in health care, business, or any of the social sciences for investments of a similar order of magnitude. From a practical perspective, the quality of evidence is certainly good enough for a business executive trying to determine if health promotion is a good investment.

Does this mean we rest on our laurels? Should we stop conducting research on the organizational or financial impact of workplace health promotion programs? Definitely not, but we should refocus our efforts in terms of methodology, the scope of our research outcomes, and where the research is conducted. The most important problems with health promotion research are: small number of randomized controlled designs; small sample sizes; short duration of the studies; lack of valid and reliable measurement tools; and inappropriate analyses[54]. Suggestions on how to address these problems are discussed below.

Individual employers should continue to conduct high quality evaluations of their programs, examining both the health and organizational outcomes of their programs. However, the primary focus of these evaluation efforts should shift to focus on how well the program supports the organization's mission, long-term goals, and current priorities. To the extent that these goals and priorities include containing medical care costs and enhancing productivity, those outcomes should be studied. Indeed, there was a burst of activity in the realm of measuring presenteeism in the past decade and we suspect it will continue to be an area of interest for researchers and practitioners. These individual program evaluation efforts should be upgraded to address two of the most common problems in research and evaluation: using valid and reliable measures, and using the appropriate analysis. For most employers, this will be difficult because, in a comprehensive program that includes organization level changes, the best unit of randomization will be at the organization level. Therefore, multiple organizations will be required to conduct this level of study.

The problems of small sample sizes and short duration of studies will be difficult to correct at the individual program evaluation level except with the largest employers. In examining medical care costs, study samples of at least 10,000 people are optimal to overcome analysis problems related to the volatility of the data. We also need cost data three years before and three years after the intervention. Ideally, we would like to have a situation in which the intervention is offered, withdrawn, and offered again. This type of research might be possible in a small number of very large organizations that have low turnover. These might include the United States Post Office, the military (focusing on career officers), or some of the twenty or so largest employers. However, this type of evaluation will be very difficult for most employers.

Even with the largest employers, it will be difficult to justify the high cost of high quality research. It is not unusual for a well-conducted study on the impact of a health promotion program on medical care utilization to cost $100,000 - $250,000 or more. Also, structuring a program to comply with research requirements might create significant delays in program implementation, causing resentment from the people not having access to the program. All of these extra problems and costs would serve no direct purpose to the employer as they already have sufficient data to show them the program can produce positive financial returns.

Another problem is the absence of a clear **temporal mechanism** to explain the link between health risks and medical care costs. For example, we would expect that people who have risk factors such as hypertension, excess stress, sedentary lifestyle, tobacco use, poor nutrition, and alcohol abuse to have higher medical care costs. However, it is reasonable to expect a lag of several years between the onset of these diseases and the increase in costs and between the elimination of the risk factor and a reduction in costs. If this lag time does exist, how should we interpret a reduction in medical care costs that occurs immediately after a health promotion program occurs? It would be reasonable to expect rapid cost reductions from programs in medical selfcare, seat belt use safety programs, and substance abuse treatment, but not in most of the other areas. For example, Musich et al. estimated that costs of former smokers returned to costs of non-smokers in five years for those with no chronic conditions and in 10 years for those with chronic conditions[89]. To fully understand the potential of health promotion programs to reduce costs, we need to conduct **longitudinal studies**.

To address the problems of study design, sample size, and duration of study, we need to create collaborative efforts among employers, private research foundations, and such government agencies as the National Institutes of Health, Centers for Disease Control and Prevention, Department of Commerce, or Department of Labor, to design, implement, and fund large scale research studies. The Health Enhancement Research Organization[90] and the American Journal of Health Promotion[91] made some progress in stimulating these efforts, but much work remains to be done. The results of these proposed studies would help set government policy, not necessarily to advise individual employers. This research might focus on producing standardized outcome measures and identifying a) which interventions are best in producing savings, b) characteristics of the most successful programs, c) how to improve the cost effectiveness of programs, and d) how to reach different gender, ethnic, and income groups.

HOW CAN AN EMPLOYER DETERMINE IF A HEALTH PROMOTION PROGRAM WILL BE A GOOD INVESTMENT?

A process is described below to help a manager determine if the program is likely to produce sufficient returns to justify its cost.

Cost/Benefit Analysis Projections

Like any other program in the organization, the health promotion program should not be a frill. It should pay for itself in terms of the benefits it brings to the organization. Some of these benefits will be tangible and measurable, such as reduced medical care costs or reduced absenteeism. Others will be more difficult to measure but equally valuable, such as improved image. Projecting the financial returns a program may generate is not simple, but it can be done and should be done as part of the **feasibility study** to determine if the program is a good investment for the organization. A "**macro-approach**" to cost/benefit analysis is described below[4]. The macro approach has seven basic steps that are also listed in Table 16.

Step 1: Identify and Quantify the Areas Affected by the Health Promotion Program

The first step in the prospective cost/benefit analysis is to determine the areas of the organization that are likely to be affected by the health promotion program, identify sources of information on each of these areas, and quantify these areas. Identifying areas that may be affected by the health promotion program will be relatively easy. A sample list of these is shown in Table 17. However, in most organizations, identifying good sources of this information and securing accurate values will be difficult. For example, many organizations track absenteeism at the department level but may not keep central records for the entire organization. Collecting data will often require a request from each department. This can be very cumbersome in an organization that has a large number of departments located in multiple geographic sites and can easily result in missing data from some departments. In some cases, absenteeism is tracked for hourly workers but not for salary workers. Other productivity related data, especially how much high quality work an employee completes per week, month, or year, is just not available in most organizations.

Collecting information on medical care spending is equally difficult. Surprisingly, even moderately large employers sometimes have trouble determining their annual medical care costs. In most cases they will know exactly how much they have paid a specific carrier, such as Blue Cross/Blue Shield, but their payments may not correspond to a specific calendar year. In other cases they may have additional commercial carriers, different carriers for active employees and retirees, and a number of HMOs, all using different calendar years for collecting premiums. This is not to say that the director of benefits could not come up with an accurate measure of current annual medical care costs if given such a directive by the president of the organization. However, it might be difficult to justify this much effort merely to provide information to facilitate a prospective cost/benefit analysis for a health promotion program. In most cases, the compilation of these figures will be left to the person conducting the study, and it is very easy to make mistakes in such compilations. This problem is compounded when collecting information on past years. This whole process is very time-consuming and subject to error due to missing or misinterpreted documents. Collecting information on productivity and image are, of course, far more difficult because most organizations do not keep information on these areas.

Step 2: Estimate the Cost Ranges of the Health Promotion Program

The next step is to determine the probable cost of the health promotion program. This may seem difficult to do before the program is fully defined, but in reality it is not difficult to project general ranges. For example, in the year 2010, the annual costs of an **awareness level** program would be between $20 and $70 per employee: a **behavior-change program** $60 to $150, including staffing; and a **comprehensive supportive-environment program** $150 to $350. During the design process, the principal designers often have a good general sense of the level of program and spending that is likely to be approved.

Step 3: Determine the Percentage Savings Required in the Areas to be affected in Order to pay for the Program

Determining the level of spending required for the program to pay for itself can be done by dividing the expenditures in the areas expected to be affected by the program by the cost of the program. For example, if annual medical care costs are $6,000 per covered life and the program is expected to cost $150 per life, the program must reduce medical care costs (or moderate future increases) by 2.50% to pay for itself ($150 ÷ $6000 = .025). Similarly, if the average employee is paid $25 per hour or $50,000 per year, the program would need to reduce paid staff time by 0.3% to pay for itself ($150 ÷ $50,000 = .003). (Paid staff time might be reduced by enhancing productivity or reducing absenteeism during hours worked. This is a very simple example used for illustrative purposes only.) Of course, if benefits are realized in both areas, the effect required in each would be reduced.

Step 4: Ask if it is Reasonable to Achieve the Level of Savings Required to Pay for the Program.

When determining whether the level of savings required to pay for the programs is reasonable if done right, the key is to ask the question not of the analyst or the health promotion expert but of the person(s) authorizing or paying for the program. This question should be asked twice. First, as part of a feasibility study senior managers should be asked to project in very rough terms how much they expect a health promotion program to affect the three major benefit areas: medical care costs, productivity, and image. Second, after the three steps above have been completed and a basic program plan has been developed, the senior executive should be shown his or her earlier estimate and the amount of savings required and asked if that level of savings seems reasonable at a gut level. The analyst can support this process by supplying research articles and answering any questions asked. The analyst should not be the one to answer the central question about whether the required savings are reasonable to achieve.

Step 5: Add Other Nonquantifiable Benefits

Some of the expected benefits will not be quantifiable, yet will be very important. For example, if the health promotion program provides an important publicity angle for the employer that is felt to be an important part of an overall image campaign, the program will provide a benefit that is very hard to quantify but is nevertheless important. Including such non-quantifiable benefits will be "frosting on the cake" if the quantifiable benefits show that the program makes sense; it may provide the necessary additional return if the quantifiable benefits are borderline.

Step 6: Compare Costs to Other Expenditures

Comparing the cost of the health promotion program to other expenditures helps the organization do a comparative **cost-effectiveness analysis** by considering how much benefit is received from current expenditures compared to those expected from the health promotion program. It is often useful to compare the program costs to each of the other employee benefits, such as paid vacation and holiday time; medical, disability, and life insurance; retirement benefits; and any subsidies for cafeterias, parking, club memberships, and other benefits. Comparing it to in-house training costs, tuition reimbursement, and out-of-town seminars helps to put these costs in perspective with other employee development costs. Comparing it to the cost of preventive maintenance and service for equipment and facilities allows developers to ask how much should be spent keeping employees in good working order as compared to equipment and facilities. Finally, it is often useful to identify all the annual expenditures of similar magnitude to the proposed health promotion program in order to allow direct comparison of the perceived benefits of these expenditures relative to the expected benefits of the health promotion program. In most cases such comparisons illustrate the relatively low cost of a health promotion program.

Step 7: Decide Whether the Program is a Good Investment

The final step, deciding whether the program is a good investment, is relatively easy if the first six steps are followed. This macro-approach provides a level of detail and sophistication that is acceptable to most business decision-makers. Although it is conceptually simple, it is a challenge to implement due to the difficulty of securing accurate information on the organization's financial expenditures.

Table 16.

Steps in Determining Whether a Health Promotion Program Is a Good Investment

Step 1:	Identify and quantify the areas affected by the health promotion program.
Step 2:	Estimate the cost ranges of the health promotion program.
Step 3:	Determine the percentage savings required in the areas to be affected in order to Pay for the program.
Step 4:	Ask if it is reasonable to achieve the level of savings required to pay for the program.
Step 5:	Add other nonquantifiable benefits.
Step 6:	Compare costs to other expenditures.
Step 7:	Decide whether the program is a good investment.

Table 17.

Areas That May be Affected by a Health Promotion Program

Impact Area	Source of Data
Productivity-related	
Absenteeism	Personnel records
Desire to work	Employee satisfaction surveys
Morale	Employee satisfaction surveys
Output per unit of time	Specialized studies
Physical and emotional disabilities	Personnel records
Recruiting success	Interviews with employment representatives
Turnover	Personnel records
Health-related	
Life insurance costs	Benefits records
Medical care costs	Personnel records
Other insurance costs	Benefits records
Type of medical claims	Medical utilization records
Worker's compensation claims	Personnel records
External Image-related	
Community	
–Current client's perceptions	Public relations department
–Potential client's perceptions	Public relations department
–Potential employee's perceptions	Public relations department
Product sales	
–Health promotion programs	Marketing department
–Other products	Marketing department

Conclusion

Keeping employees healthy is very important to most employers, and this is the reason most frequently cited by top managers for developing health promotion programs. Many top managers will fund a program because they want to keep employees healthy and because it is "the right thing to do." However, few programs will survive or thrive on a long-term basis unless they contribute to the mission, long-term goals, and short-term priorities of the organization, or to the special interests of those who approve program budgets AND top management sees data on a regular basis that shows the connection between the program and those organizational outcomes.

The most common justification for health promotion programs is medical care cost containment. A persuasive body of research has emerged that shows that people with unhealthy lifestyles do cost more and that health promotion programs can produce savings in excess of their costs. However, saving money through medical care cost containment will be important to employers only when medical care costs are perceived to be a serious problem.

Returns from productivity related outcomes including enhancing morale, reducing absenteeism, attracting and retaining good employees, and making sure that employees are physically and emotionally able to work are likely to be far greater than returns from medical care cost savings. These areas are also more likely to be closely related to the mission, longterm goals, and short-term priorities of the organization. Research examining the relationship between health promotion programs and productivity does show that programs are associated with reduced absenteeism, and that the returns from absenteeism are greater than the returns from medical care cost containment when compared from a cost/benefit perspective. Predictions by the authors that this would be a rapidly growing area of research did not come true, probably because of the challenges in conducting this research.[92]

Research or program evaluation on the impact of health promotion programs on medical care costs or productivity is expensive to conduct for most employers. Therefore, most employers must rely on research conducted in other organizations and extrapolate those findings to their own employees. Furthermore, this research or program evaluation is very difficult to execute, and few if any studies have been able to eliminate all of the methodological problems.

Nevertheless, for the field in general, the data supporting the claim that health promotion programs can reduce medical care costs and reduce absenteeism is of higher quality than the data most businesses have to support other investments of similar cost and thus is adequate to justify an investment in a health promotion program. A protocol is described here which shows how employers can decide if a health promotion program is likely to produce a positive return for their organization without conducting expensive research or making precise assumptions about financial returns.

Program managers trying to justify their programs will probably be most successful if they determine the mission, long-term goals, short-term priorities of their organization, and the special interests of those who approve program budgets, THEN design their programs to enhance these organizational outcomes. Next, they should design their program evaluation plan to measure the impact of the program on these outcomes, and make sure top management sees those data on a regular basis.

References

1   Kaiser Family Foundation and Health Research and Educational Trust. *Employer Health Benefits: 2012 Annual Survey.* Menlo Park, CA. 2012.

2   Association for Worksite Health Promotion, U.S. Department of Health and Human Services, William M. Mercer, Inc. *1999 National worksite health promotion survey.* Northbrook, IL: Association for Worksite Health Promotion and William M. Mercer, Inc. 2000.

3   U.S. Department of Health and Human Services. Healthy People 2020: healthy people in healthy communities. ODPHP Publication Number B0132. Washington, D.C. 2010.

4   MetLife. 10th Annual Study of Employee Benefits Trends. New York, NY, 2012.

5   Linnan L, Bowling M, Childress J, Lindsay G, Blakey C, Pronk S, Wieker S, Royall P. Results of the 2004 national worksite health promotion survey. *Am J Pub Health.* 2008;98:1503-1509.

6   Department of Health and Human Services, Public Health Service. 1992 National survey of worksite health promotion activities: Summary. *Am J Health Promot. 1993;*7(6):452-464.

7   O'Donnell M, Harris J. Health Promotion in the Workplace (2nd ed.). Albany, NY: Delmar Publishers. 1994.

8   Goetzel R, Ozminkowski R. What's Holding You Back: Why Should (or Shouldn't) Employers Invest in Health Promotion Programs for Their Workers? *N Car Med J.* 2006;67:428-430.

9   O'Donnell M, Bishop C, Kaplan K. Benchmarking best practices in workplace health promotion. *Art Health Promot.* 1997;1:1.

10 European Foundation for the Improvement of Living and Working Conditions. *Workplace Health Promotion in Europe: Programme Summary.* Dublin, Ireland. 1997.

11 European Agency for Safety and Health at Work. *Motivation for employers to carry out workplace health promotion.* Publications Office of the European Union, Luxembourg. 2012.

12   Organization for Economic Cooperation and Development. OECD Health Data 2012 - Frequently Requested Data. Paris, France. 2012.

13   Centers for Medicaid and Medicare Services. *National Health Expenditure Data*. Baltimore, MD. 2011.

14   Levit K, Cowan C. The burden of health care costs: Business, household, government. *Health Care Fin Rev.* 1990;12(2):131.

15   Koretz G. Employers tame medical costs: But workers pick up a bigger share. *Bus Week*, January 17, 2000, p. 26.

16   Interstudy. The Interstudy Competitive Edge: HMO Industry Report, 9.1. Bloomington, MN: InterStudy Publications. 1999.

17   Hoechst Marion Roussell, *HMO/PPO/Medicare-Medicaid Digest*. Kansas City: MO; 1999.

18   Health Care Financing Administration. National Health Care Expenditures, 2000. Washington DC.

19   William M. Mercer, Inc. 14th Annual National Survey of Employer-Sponsored Health Plans. 2000. Northbrook, IL.

20   Finkelstein A. The aggregate effects of health insurance: evidence from the introduction of Medicare. *Q J of Econ.* 2007;122(1):1-37.

21   Haviland AM, Marquis MS, McDevitt R, Sood N. Growth of Consumer-Directed Health Plans to one-half of all employer-sponsored insurance could save $57 billion annually. *Health Aff.* 2012;31:1009-1015.

22   Brink S. *Health risks and behavior: The impact on medical costs*. Brookfield, WI: Millman and Robertson. 1987.

23   Yen L, Edington D, Witting P. Associations between health risk appraisal scores and employee medical claims costs. *Am J Health Promot.* 1991;6(1):46-54.

24   Yen L, Edington D, Witting P. Prediction of prospective medical claims and absenteeism costs for 1284 hourly workers from a manufacturing company. *J Occup Med.* 1992;34 (4):428-435.

25   Goetzel R. Relationship between modifiable health risks and health care expenditures. *J Occup Environ Med.* 1998;40:10.

26   Goetzel RZ, Pei X, Tabrizi MJ, Henke RM, Kowlessar N, Nelson CF, Metz RD. Ten modifiable health risk factors are linked to more than one-fifth of employer-employee health care spending. *Health Aff.* 2012;31:2474-2484.

27   Schultz AB, Edington DW. Metabolic syndrome in a workplace: prevalence, co-morbidities, and economic impact. *Met Syn Rel Disord.* 2009;7:459-468.

28   Braunstein A, Li Y, Hirschland D, McDonald T, Edington DW. Internal associations among health-risk factors and risk prevalence. *Am J Health Behav.* 2001;25:407-417.

29   Mayer JP, Taylor JR, Thrush JC. Exploratory cluster analysis of behavioral risks for chronic disease and injury: implications for tailoring health promotion services. *J Comm Health.* 1990;15:377-389.

30   Anderson DR, Whitmer RW, Goetzel RZ, Ozminkowski RJ, Dunn RL, Wasserman J, Serxner S. The relationship between modifiable health risks and group-level health care expenditures: Health Enhancement Research Organization (HERO) Research Committee. *Am J Health Promot.* 2001;15(1):45-52.

31   Jee S, O'Donnell M, Suh I, Kim I. The relationship between modifiable health risks and future medical care expenditures: the Korea Medical Insurance Corporation (KMIC) Study. *Am J Health Promot.* 2001;15(4):244-255.

32   Anderson G. Multinational comparisons of health care: Expenditures, coverage, and outcomes. New York, NY: The Commonwealth Fund; 1998.

33   Edington DW. *Zero Trends: Health as a serious economic strategy.* University of Michigan Health Management Research Center; Ann Arbor, MI. 2009.

34   Yen L, McDonald T, Hirschland D, Edington DW. Association between wellness score from a Health Risk Appraisal and prospective medical claims costs. *J Occup Environ Med.* 2003;45:1049-1057.

35   Edington D. *Worksite wellness; 20-year cost benefit analysis and report: 1979 to 1998.* Ann Arbor, MI: University of Michigan, Health Management Research Center. 1998.

36   Steinwachs DM. Pharmacy benefit plans and prescription drug spending. *JAMA*. 2002;288: 1773-1774.

37   Levit K, Cowan C, Lazenby H, Sensenig A, McDonnell P, Stiller J, Martin A, Health Accounts Team. Health spending in 1998: signals of changes. *Health Aff*. 2000;19:124-132.

38   Milliman. 2012 Milliman Medical Index. Seattle, WA. 2012.

39   Yen L, Schultz AB, Schnueringer E, Edington DW. Financial costs due to excess health risks among active employees of a utility company. *J Occup Environ Med*. 2006;48:896-905.

40   Burton WN, Chen CY, Conti DJ, Schultz AB, Edington DW. Measuring the relationship between employees' health risk factors and corporate pharmaceutical expenditures. *J Occup Environ Med*. 2003;45:793-802.

41   Edington DW, Yen LT, Witting P. The financial impact of changes in personal health practices. *J Occup Environ Med*. 1997;39:1037-1046.

42   Edington DW, Musich S. Associating changes in health risk levels with changes in medical and short-term disability costs. *Health and Productivity Management*. 2004;3[1]:12-15.

43   Schultz AB, Edington DW. The association between changes in metabolic syndrome and changes in cost in a workplace population. *J Occup Environ Med*. 2009;51:771-779.

44   Edington DW. Emerging research: a view from one research center. *Am J Health Promot*. 2001;15:341-349.

45   Nyce S, Grossmeier J, Anderson DR, Terry PE, Kelley B. Association between changes in health risk status and changes in future health care costs. *J Occup Environ Med*. 2012; 54:1364-1376.

46   Pelletier K. A review and analysis of the health and cost effectiveness outcome studies of comprehensive health promotion and disease prevention programs at the worksite. *Am J Health Promot*. 1991;5:311-315.

47   Pelletier K. A review and analysis of the health and cost effectiveness outcome studies of comprehensive health promotion and disease prevention programs at the worksite, 1991-1993 Update. *Am J Health Promot*. 1993;8:43-49.

48   Pelletier K. A review and analysis of the health and cost effectiveness outcome studies of comprehensive health promotion and disease prevention programs at the worksite, 1993–1995 Update. *Am J Health Promot.* 1996;10:380-388.

49   Pelletier K. A review and analysis of the health and cost effectiveness outcome studies of comprehensive health promotion and disease prevention programs at the worksite, 1995-1998 Update. *Am J Health Promot.* 1999;13(5),66-78.

50   Pelletier K. A review and analysis of the health and cost-effectiveness studies of comprehensive health promotion and disease management programs at the worksite: 1998-2000 Update. *Am J Health Promot.* 2001;16(2):107-116.

51   Pelletier K. A review and analysis of the clinical and cost-effectiveness studies of comprehensive health promotion and disease management programs at the worksite: update VI 2000-2004. *J Occup Environ Med.* 2005;47:1051-1058.

52   Pelletier K. A review and analysis of the clinical and cost-effectiveness studies of comprehensive health promotion and disease management programs at the worksite: Update VII 2004-2008. *J Occup Environ Med.* 2009;51:822-837.

53   Loeppke R, Edington DW, Beg S. Impact of the Prevention Plan on employee health risk reduction. *Pop Health Mgmt.* 2010;13:275-284.

54   Aldana S. Financial impact of worksite health promotion and methodological quality of the evidence. *Art Health Promot.* 1998;2(1):1-8.

55   Aldana S. Financial impact of health promotion programs: a comprehensive review of the literature. *Am J Health Promot.* 2001;15(5):296-320.

56   Chapman LS. Meta-evaluation of worksite health promotion economic return studies. *Am J Health Promot.* 2003;17(3):1-10.

57   Chapman LS. Meta-evaluation of worksite health promotion economic return studies. *Am J Health Promot.* 2005;19(6):1-10.

58   Chapman LS. Meta-evaluation of worksite health promotion economic return studies: 2012 update. *Am J Health Promot* 2012;26(4):1-12.

59   Baicker KM, Cutler D, Song Z. Workplace wellness programs can generate savings. *Health Aff.* 2010;29:304-311.

60 Edington DW. Changes in costs related to changes in psychological and social support risk factors. Paper presented at Art and Science of Health Promotion Conference, Colorado Springs, Colorado. 2000.

61 Aldana S, Pronk NP. Health promotion programs, modifiable health risks, and employee absenteeism. *J Occup Environ Med.* 2001;43:36-46.

62 Serxner S, Gold DB, Bultman KK. The impact of behavioral health risks on worker absenteeism. *J Occup Environ Med.* 2001;43:347-354.

63 Musich S, Napier D, Edington DW. The association of health risks with workers' compensation costs. *J Occup Environ Med.* 2001;43:534-541.

64 Wright DW, Beard MJ, Edington DW. Association of health risks with the cost of time away from work. *J Occup Environ Med.* 2002;44:1126-1134.

65 Kuhnen AE, Burch SP, Shenolikar RA, Joy KA. Employee health and frequency of workers' compensation and disability claims. *J Occup Environ Med.* 2009;51:1041-1048.

66 International Labor Organization. *Key Indicators of the Labour Market.* Geneva, Switzerland. 2011.

67 U.S. Department of Commerce, Bureau of Economic Analysis. Gross Domestic Product. 2012. Available at http://www.bea.gov. Accessed March 2013.

68 Johns G. Presenteeism in the workplace: a review and research agenda. *J Org Behav.* 2009;31:519-542.

69 Mattke S, Balakrishnan A, Bergamo G, Newberry SJ. A review of methods to measure health-related productivity loss. *Am J Manag Care.* 2007;13:211-217.

70 Schultz AB, Edington DW. Employee health and presenteeism: a systematic review. *J Occup Rehab.* 2007;17:547-579.

71 Lofland JH, Pizzi L, Frick KD. A review of health-related workplace productivity loss instruments. *Pharmacoeconomics.* 2004;22:165-184.

72 Burton WN, Conti DJ, Chen CY, Schultz AB, Edington DW. The role of health risk factors and disease on worker productivity. *J Occup Environ Med.* 1999;41:863-877.

[73] Brooks A, Hagen SE, Sathyanarayanan S, Schultz AB, Edington DW Presenteeism: critical issues. *J Occup Environ Med.* 2010;52:1055-1067.

[74] Cyr A, Hagen S. Measurement and quantification of presenteeism: letters to the editor. *J Occup Environ Med.* 2007;50:163-171.

[75] Pelletier B, Boles M, Lynch W. Change in health risks and work productivity over time. *J Occup Environ Med.* 2004;46:746-754.

[76] Burton WN, Chen CY, Conti DJ, Schultz AB, Edington DW. The association between health risk change and presenteeism change. *J Occup Environ Med.* 2006;48:252-263.

[77] Mills PR, Kessler RC, Cooper J, Sullivan S. Impact of a health promotion program on employee health risks and work productivity. *Am J Health Promot.* 2007;22:45-53.

[78] Loeppke R. The value of health and the power of prevention. *Int J Workplace Health Mgmt.* 2008;1:95-108.

[79] Towers Watson/National Business Group on Health. Performance in an era of uncertainty: 17th annual employer survey on purchasing value in health care. New York, NY. 2012.

[80] American Hospital Association. A Call to Action: Creating a Culture of Health. http://www.aha.org/aha/issues/Health-for-life/culture.html. Accessed April 5, 2013.

[81] Kerwin K, Treece J. Detroit's big chance: Can it regain business and respect it lost in the past 20 years? *Bus Week*, June 29, 1992, p. 82.

[82] Green L, Cargo M. The future of health promotion. In M. O'Donnell & J. Harris (Eds.) Health Promotion in the Workplace (2nd ed.,pp. 497-524). Albany, NY: Delmar Publishers. 1994.

[83] Grossmeier J, Terry PE, Cipriotti A, Burtaine JE. Best practices in evaluating worksite health promotion programs. *Art Health Promot.* 2010. 12(1):1-9.

[84] Wolf R, Slack T, Rose-Hearn T. Factors influencing the adoption and maintenance of Canadian facilities-based worksite health promotion programs. *Am J Health Promot.* 1993;7:189-198.

[85] Goetzel R, Ozminkowski R. The health and cost benefits of worksite health promotion pro-grams. *Ann Rev Pub Health*. 2008;29:303-323.

[86] Bertera R. The effects of behavioral risks on absenteeism and health care costs in the workplace. *J Occup Med*. 1991;33,1119-1124.

[87] Goetzel R, Juday T, Ozminkowski R. What's the ROI? A systematic review of return on in-vestment studies of corporate health and productivity management initiatives. *Worksite Health*. 1999;6(3):12-21.

[88] Conrad K, Conrad K, Walcott-McQuigg J. Threats to internal validity in worksite health promotion program research: Common problems and possible solutions. *Am J Health Promot*. 1991;6,112-222.

[89] Musich S. Faruzzi SD, Lu C, McDonald T, Hirschland D, Edington DW Pattern of Medical Charges After Quitting Smoking Among Those With and Without Arthritis, Allergies, or Back Pain. *Am J Health Promot*. 2003; 18:133-142.

[90] O'Donnell M, Whitmer W, Anderson D. Is it time for a national health promotion research agenda? *Am J Health Promot*. 1999;13:3.

[91] O'Donnell M. Editor 's Notes: Building health promotion into the national agenda. *Am J Health Promot*. 2000;14:3.

[92] O'Donnell MP. Health Promotion in the Workplace. 3rd ed. Albany, NY: Cenage, 2002.

About the Author

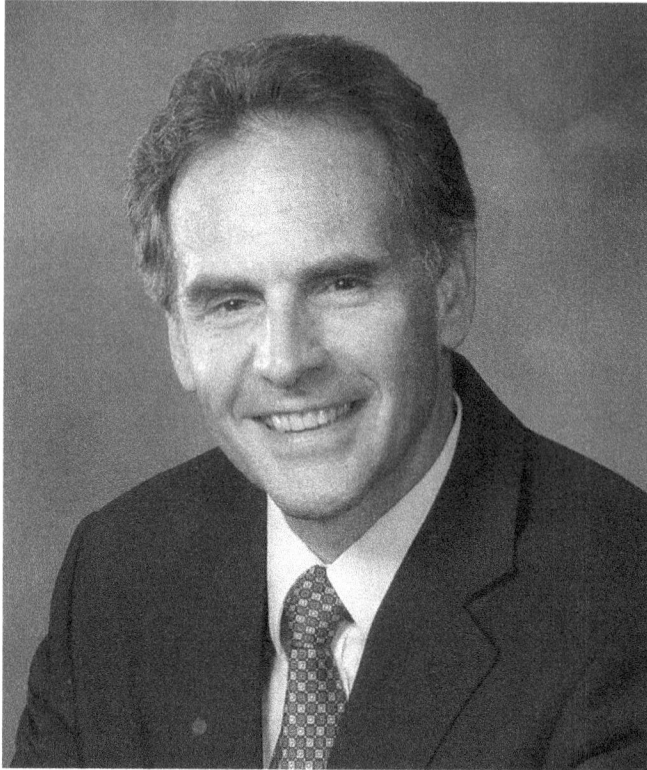

Dr. O'Donnell is the Director of the Health Management Research Center in the School of Kinesiology of the University of Michigan. Formed in 1978, the Center has helped more than 1000 worksites measure the health risks of their employees; calculate the link between health risks, medical costs and productivity; evaluate the impact of their health promotion programs; and in the process, establish the scientific foundation for this area of research. Dr. O'Donnell has worked directly with employers, health care organizations, government agencies, foundations, insurance companies and health promotion providers to develop new and refine existing health promotion programs and has served in leadership roles in four major health systems. He is Founder, President and Editor-in-Chief of the *American Journal of Health Promotion* and is also Founder and Chairman Emeritus of Health Promotion Advocates, a non-profit policy group created to integrate health promotion strategies into national policy. Health Promotion Advocates was successful in developing six provisions that became law as part of the Affordable Care Act. He has co-authored 6 books and workbooks, including *Health Promotion in the Workplace*, which was in continuous publication for 27 years, and more than 190 articles, book chapters and columns. He has presented more than 260 keynote and workshop presentations on six continents, served on boards and committees for 48 non-profit and for-profit organizations and received 13 national awards. His most recent awards are the Elizabeth Fries Health Education Award presented by the James F. and Sarah T. Fries Foundation, and the Bill WhitmerLeadership Award, presented by the Health Enhancement Research Organization (HERO). He earned a PhD in Health Behavior from University of Michigan, an MBA in General Management and an MPH in Hospital Management, both from University of California, Berkeley, and an AB in psychobiology from Oberlin College. He attended high school and was later a Senior Fulbright Scholar and visiting professor in Seoul, South Korea.